How To Groon  Beginners 2023

Comprehensive Modern Guide To Grooming Your Pet Dog: Cleaning, Brushing And Healthy Care

Mark Stilwell

Copyright©2022 **Mark Stilwell**

All Rights Reserved

TABLE OF CONTENT

Introduction..3

Chapter 1 simple procedures for cleaning a dog's nails,ear and teeth...4

Chapter 2 Basic tools and equipment for grooming dog..24

Chapter 3 Do not trim a dirty or matted coat...............27

Chapter 4 What You Need To Know To Handle Matted Dog Hair..30

Chapter 5 Take Fluffy for a bath................................37

Chapter 6 Pay attention to your dog's temperament and health..48

Chapter 7 vaccination as a way of grooming a dog......55

Chapter 8 conclusion…………………………………………….69

INTRODUCTION

Regular dog grooming is essential to preserving your companion dog's happiness and physical health. Since grooming unquestionably entails giving your dog a bath or brushing, all you need are the necessary tools and equipment on hand to take care of your dog. Teeth, ears, and nail washing are also included. Additionally, it would be best if you were prepared to handle any other problem, including matted hair and skunk spray.

CHAPTER ONE

Simple procedures for cleaning a dogs nails,ear and teeth.

This post will provide you with some quick and straightforward advice for taking care of your dog's teeth, ears, and nails.

You might respond, "But I have my vet and my groomer for that."

That is one perspective, but hiring someone to give you this kind of care will cost you money that you could easily save if you did it yourself.

Additionally, having other people handle our pets in these temperate regions can be highly traumatic for them.

They are more likely to trust you and feel at ease with you if you do it. Thus it is better for you.

What we do is as follows.

Your dog's ears: Prevent future significant issues...

Here is a detailed cleaning schedule.

You may not be aware of it, but you should schedule frequent ear exams on your calendar.

It may be daily for some dogs, weekly for others, or monthly for still others. You won't honestly know until you check your dog's ears to see how frequently they become dirty and require cleaning.

And cleaning could entail using a natural cleaning solution or just a few cotton swabs. Just clear out what you can see without digging too far. A headlight is used to aid humans.

If you discover that you require more than a cotton swab, consider the following natural cleaning method:

Three tablespoons of hydrogen peroxide, one tablespoon of apple cider vinegar, and 1/3 cup witch hazel;

The solution can be kept in a cold, dry area.

Dunk it into the cotton swab to use. Use a small amount; avoid over-saturation.

And for particular ear disorders, think about including the following:

Add colloidal silver to treat ear infections, oregano oil to treat yeasty ears, lavender to soothe inflamed ears, and neem oil to treat ear mites.

If your eardrum has ruptured, avoid using any cleaning.

What if your dog doesn't like it when you poke around in its ears?

However, it would help if you first accustomed them to it, and the optimum time to do it is when they are still young puppies. They'll become much more accustomed to it the more often you do it.

But if you maintain a regular routine, even grownups will acclimate to it.

The simplest methods we've discovered for maintaining our dog's teeth in excellent condition.

Teeth problems are frequently caused by our pets' processed and dry meals. That means spending more of our hard-earned money on routine dental care for them while also going through the stress of putting our beloved canines under anaesthesia for a potentially dangerous treatment.

Is it preferable to give our dogs a diet consisting solely of raw animal products, as this would prevent them from developing dental problems?

We can confirm that feeding our dogs just raw food has improved their dental health, and once we figured out how to do it, we were astounded by how simple it is to do so. From our video instruction, available here, you may learn more about providing raw food to your dog.

However, even if we feed our dogs raw food, we still need to take two extra steps to maintain healthy teeth.

While you could attempt to brush your dog's teeth alone, we know that most people won't make the time. We comprehend! Building cooperation needs patience and experience. Additionally, the brushing that does take place probably won't be beneficial if your dog has not been trained to participate.

This all-natural product produced from seaweed, which we incorporate daily in their meals, is helpful. Look at it here.

The second thing we do is give them large raw (never cooked) meaty bones to chew on. These come directly from the ranchers from whom we buy the meat for our meals and the dog food products we offer.

However, they must be substantial. Knucklebones that are difficult for them to grasp. Avoid purchasing anything little that they could swallow whole, split apart, or wrap their entire jaw around. The bones should be large enough for them to nibble on but not bite. Their risk of shattering and cracking teeth increases when they can wrap their jaw around anything hard, such as bones or antlers.

The majority of commercial chew goods are not something we advise using since not only are they processed, but dogs can choke on them and may swallow parts that they later vomit back up on your carpet or couch.

Like humans, though, we cannot overstate the importance of food in maintaining healthy teeth. Give your dogs the raw food they were designed to consume. Avoid eating commercial dry foods. The remainder of providing kids with healthy teeth then becomes much more straightforward.

How to clip dog nails quickly

When we tell people that grooming my dogs' nails is drama-free, quick, and requires no restraint, many of them are in awe.

You wonder if that's feasible. Absolutely, it is!

The only restraint necessary is to hold their paws still while we use the nail clipper to trim their nails. We have worked hard to ensure nail trimmings are simple, as stress-free as possible, and require no other restraint.

And now for the secret...

Consistent practice, please!

How do we interpret that?

We scheduled a time to at least cut my dogs' nails every other week on our calendar. It has been a habit for us because we do it so frequently and have been doing it since we first got my dogs, but more importantly, it has become a habit for our dogs.

It can take time for you to train your dog to accept it, but if you schedule it each week, we promise it will happen.

The alternative, which is frequently insufficient, is to have your pet's veterinarian or groomer do it sometimes.

First, because nails develop just like human nails do, it is crucial to check and trim nails frequently. Do you want to take your dog to the vet or a groomer to get their nails trimmed every few weeks? We don't have the time or money, so that's okay with you.

Second, we've seen what might happen when groomers or veterinary offices must hold and muzzle dogs to clip their nails. Every time, they get more complicated, and for some dogs, the stress is too much.

How can you cut your dog's nails fast, efficiently, and with the least stress while saving money because you are doing it yourself?

We appreciate your inquiry.

What we do is as follows:

1. Begin by teaching your dogs to lie on their side. (Or, if it's more convenient, to hold another position.) Include this crucial "trick" in your training regimen. Sue teaches this in some of her classes and in her online course on dog training. View the how-to video right here. The process is straightforward. Reward your dog for acting repeatedly. By postponing their reward, be sure to gradually add more extended periods for them to hold this stance.

2. You should practice handling your dog simultaneously so that they become accustomed to your touching them. Handle them frequently and examine their paws and

nails. Your dog will get used to you doing that with this aid.

3. Get your dog to lay down in the position you taught them, then gently trim the tips of their nails while they maintain the down-on-the-side position. If it is simpler to have someone else feed while you clip nails, you can enlist some assistance.

4. To start, you should break up your nail-trimming sessions and focus on just one foot or even just one nail at a time. Then, you can come back later to finish the other. Be patient since you must train your dog to become accustomed to these sessions. Start with brief sessions, as Sue suggests in her training.

Your dog will become used to it more if you follow the advice above and are consistent. Some dogs adjust to it right away, while others need more time.

While some individuals think a dremmel is preferable, clippers are the most excellent instrument for the job. If you use a dremmel, be sure to help your dog get used to the sound before using it on the nails because the vibration and noise can be distressing for some dogs. We found using nail clippers to be a lot simpler.

Ask your groomer or a veterinary technician to show you the proper technique if you need help knowing how to clip your own nails. Even if you feel you can't do it yourself, following these instructions will make it much simpler for your groomer or vet tech to perform the actual trims. They'll be grateful that you did!

1. Begin with the nails

Giving your dog frequent nail trims every few weeks, even if it's not a duty either of you particularly loves, is one of the essential stages for keeping them groomed at home. While some dogs' nails may naturally grow shorter when walking on concrete or other hard surfaces, some need regular nail clipping.

Most pet retailers carry nail clippers in various diameters to fit different dog breeds. "A good time to trim them is once every four to six weeks." A dab of cornstarch or styptic powder will stop the bleeding if you accidentally nick the "quick," which are the nerves and blood vessels inside the nail, which some dogs have on the side of their feet.

Both you and your dog may experience anxiety while having their nails cut. However, guessing where to clip their nails is OK to prevent injury. The dog groomers at Canine to Five in Detroit have created the ideal at-home manual for clipping your dog's nails, which will take you through the process step-by-step.

How do I use it?

Not all nail trimmers are created equal, so choosing the right one for your dog's breed and size can help you succeed.

Scissor-style clippers are required for small dogs or tiny puppies.

When to trim?

As soon as your dog's nails begin touching the ground, it would be best to clip them. A dog's nails will continue to grow until they curl outward, or worse, inward, just like human nails do. Long nails can be painful for your dog to walk on, they reduce your dog's traction, they're more likely to break or entirely fall off, and they can grow into your dog's paw pads, causing pain and infection. It might be time for a nail trim if you hear your dog's nails clicking on the ground.

How should I trim?

The most significant query is WHERE? Most dog owners are aware that a dog's nail contains a vein known as the quick. The source of both your blood and your anxiety is one vein. If you're lucky—and yes, you can genuinely get lucky when it comes to dog nails—your dog will have white or clear nails that allow you to see the quick from the outside.

The quick cannot be seen from the exterior of the nail for many of us because our dogs either have one or more nails that are entirely black. The best course of action in this situation is to trim gradually, as discussed in the section after.

How do you trim?

Now that we know what to use, when, and where to cut it, what technique is the most effective? If you're clipping your dog's nails for the first time or you already know they get a little anxious while getting a pedicure, start by including some positive reinforcement training. This video demonstrates how to desensitize your dog to the thought of having their nails cut and turn it into a pleasant experience for them.

Do keep some important parts clipped.

Starting by dry-trimming only the most required places if you want to prolong the life of an existing cut or maybe need more time to be ready to undertake a thorough groom yourself. According to Minaker, "the face, ears, and sanitary areas should be maintained." It can assist with odour and avoid infection to keep the hair short and clean in these areas, and you don't need to use good grooming scissors for this type of trim. As long as the scissors are reasonably sharp and haven't been used for anything else, Minaker advises using decent craft scissors.

CHAPTER TWO

Basic tools and equipment for grooming dog

Do purchase a grooming set.

Purchase a pet clipper or grooming kit with multiple blades if you wish to trim your dog's entire body. Become comfortable using the equipment; it might take some time and practice. The instructions to find out what kind of blade to use and how short to trim your dog's hair. And don't worry about purchasing a pricey clipper unless you intend to continue doing this frequently.

You undoubtedly want your pet to look, feel, and smell its best if you own a dog. If you live in a big city, going to the spa once a month (or more frequently if your dog enjoys playing in the mud) can be time-consuming and expensive. Instead, why not buy some quality dog grooming supplies and do it yourself at home? Depending on your dog's breed, fur type, and temperament, the best dog grooming kit will spoil them while saving you money and time getting about. With this dog grooming equipment in your possession, you can soon win over your dog's love for you as a groomer and his love for you as a parent.ConairPro 5-Piece Starter Kit is the best beginner kit. HANSPROU Dog Shaver Clippers are the best essential clippers. oneisall Dog Grooming Kit is the best cordless clipper. Professional Animal Grooming Clippers are the best dog grooming investment. Outram Grooming Kit is the best budget option.

Chapter three

Do not trim a dirty or matted coat.

"The first step is to ensure the dog is well groomed – many people are unaware that a dog should be brushed before it is showered. There will be twice as much of a nightmare if there is any matting and the coat is not brushed out. Depending on your dog's hair, you can use different brushes or combs; a wide-tooth comb is suggested for tangles. Put your finger between the mats and the dog's skin to prevent yanking on the furs and pulling on the skin, advises Minaker. She also suggests using a small amount of pet or human hair conditioner to help with brushing.

Simple Solutions for Matted Dog Hair

The worst dog hair is matted! It's unsightly, filthy, and occasionally painful. Once matted dog hair starts, it can get out of hand and become a health problem.

I once looked after a brother-and-sister pair of Blue Picardy Spaniels. These majestic dogs' legs, bottom, and tail are covered in beautiful, wavy feathering. This breed is also very spirited! After a lengthy trek filled with romping through streams and adding that gorgeous feathered coat, you have some seriously matted dog hair.

The real stinger was that the siblings' parents insisted their fur could not be clipped. After our outside excursions, I would try to help by brushing them, but I felt awful for the groomer when I had to tell the staff, "No cutting!" when I dropped them off. Those two puppies would return with silky, mat-free feathers as if by magic. How did they handle all that matted dog hair? Patience, the proper equipment, ability, and assistance from watchful dog parents.

Dog with wild, untidy hair that blows in the wind.

CHAPTER FOUR

What You Need To Know To Handle Matted Dog Hair.

Following is some grooming advice for handling matted dog hair:

1. To get the mats out, you must first train your dog to enjoy being groomed. Even if your puppy doesn't require it, start brushing him when he is small. Give him high-value rewards and praise to help him connect grooming with positive experiences.

2. Pay close attention to areas that mat easily, such as where his collar or halter rubs, behind the ears, in the armpits, and under the undercarriage.

3. Prevent the development of dog hair mats.

Before your dog jumps into a river or lake, use a detangler cream or spray to help prevent fur from getting clumped up. This will make the post-swim brush out easier. Use only items designed exclusively for dogs.

4. Visit the vet if your pup's coat has become seriously matted or hasn't been looked after in a while. Extremely matted dog hair and an unlooked-for coat might irritate or infect the skin, necessitating medical attention.

5. Ask your groomer for advice on the best method and brush to use when brushing your dog. Your groomer will be pleased to share, as it makes her job easier the better you are at maintaining daily maintenance.

6. Pay attention to the paws.

Between the pads of the feet, hair can grow and become matted. Maintain a short haircut. Purchase some dog clippers if you feel the need to touch up between professional grooming sessions. They are less traumatic for your dog's delicate paw pads than scissors.

7. Clippers are also helpful for maintaining a dog's tidy rear end. It can quickly become dirty in that space between sitting and urinating. A little humiliation between you and your dog is worth maintaining a clean area around the anus.

8. A healthy diet enables him to have a coat that is less likely to result in matted dog hair. Check the food and supplements you give your dog for omega-3 or fish oil.

Of course, a veterinarian should be consulted to determine the ideal dosage for your dog.

How do experienced dog groomers handle matted dog hair?

1. If your dog has mats or tangled hair, never bathe him. Water makes them tighter by acting like a sponge.

2. To help untangle matted dog hair, use corn starch. Brush out after rubbing some into the mat to aid in loosening.

3. Don't rely on conditioner to get rid of or loosen mats. Before the bath, they must be carefully brushed and combed out.

4. DO NOT attempt to remove matted dog hair. You could easily cut your pet if the mats are tighter than you believe or have skin caught in them.

1. Brush! Non-shedding dogs, such as Poodles and Golden doodles, require assistance from their owners by being brushed at least twice a week with a decent slicker brush.

2. Visiting a professional groomer regularly is essential to prevent matted dog hair! It is advised to do so every six to eight weeks.

3. Rather than at the top of the hair, mats start at the base. Even though your dog may appear to have no mats, you should still run your fingers through the hair at the nape to check for tangles and snarls. It is

significantly simpler to remove a potential carpet if it is caught early.

4. Research the particular grooming requirements of your breed. Depending on your breed, different procedures will be needed to maintain a healthy and colourful coat or hair.

Three. Roomer Girls Pet Salon,

1. Whenever possible, work in small sections and work your way up to the skin from the hair's ends.

2. Consistently use quality conditioner. Even when done correctly, dematting can result in significant breakage.

3. As the final step in the tub, always rinse with cooler, warm water. The hair shafts will be sealed as a result. Warmer water opens them up, making the hair more

brittle and vulnerable to injury. Damaged and broken hair tangles more easily. Use a final conditioning spray at all times.

CHAPTER FIVE

Take Fluffy for a bath.

It's time to bathe your dog after giving them a thorough brushing. Although you could get away with using baby shampoo in a pinch.Shampoo designed expressly for dogs, more specifically "...an oatmeal and aloe shampoo because that nourishes the hair and actually helps with the scalp as well." Additionally, some shampoos target particular issues like flaky skin and hair shedding. Once your dog has been showered, towel dries them off (or blow dry them if you can), and give them another brush when their coat has completely dried. Your dog is now prepared for a trim!

How Frequently Should I Bathe My Dog?

You usually only need to bathe your dog once a month unless your pet has spent the afternoon playing about in mud puddles. Breed-specific factors come into play here; for example, longer-coated dogs may need more regular bathing or even visits to a groomer. Consult a groomer or your veterinarian if you need help with how frequently to soap up your dog. Giving a bath once a month is crucial, though.

Dogs develop an entirely new layer of skin cells every 30 days or so. "The aged cells, therefore, slough off. Dander and other similar products are produced in this way. Thus, regular grooming or bathing helps to reduce that dander.

Important Goods and Tools

Your initial choice is where you will bathe your dog. The size of your dog will likely influence your decision. A little dog might fit in the kitchen sink for a bath, but a large dog will need more room. Some pet owners like dog-specific bathtubs, whether they are standalone units, built-in units, or located in a DIY dog bath facility. Using a designated dog bath space can prevent fur and filth from blocking your family bathtub. But it's also acceptable if you want to bathe your dog in the household bathtub. Pick a location where you can bring your dog in and out of the cleaning area without risk.

Then, make sure you have all your supplies and tools close at hand before turning on the faucet.

You want to have everything you need, exactly where you can reach it." You want to avoid going around your house chasing a wet dog in search of conditioner. Of course, you'll need towels, shampoo, and conditioner on your supplies list. You may also want an eye wash and a non-slip bath mat.

Select quality shampoo and conditioner.

You need to start with the correct supplies if you want to give your dog a thorough bath. Make careful to use shampoo designed exclusively for pets. Dogs' skin has a different pH than people's. Therefore, they are more alkaline. It can irritate someone's skin if they use shampoo designed for people.

Puppy-specific shampoo may be a good idea when bathing a puppy. Puppy shampoo's pH is similar to that of a dog's eyes, so if any goes in there, it won't bother the eyes as much.

Ask a groomer what products they use if you need clarification about the ones to choose for your particular dog. Use a gentle shampoo. A shampoo to treat your dog's ailment, such as itchy skin, maybe the best option.

The crucial next step is applying a conditioner to your dog's coat after shampooing. When doing your own grooming at home, you should always follow up with a conditioner because using shampoo strips the skin and hair of many of their natural oils.your conditioner hydrates the epidermis and seals up every cell on the exterior of the hair shaft itself. "Using the conditioner is re hydrating."

Correct Dog Washing Methods

The real fun starts once you have selected the ideal location and ready-to-use supplies. Our experts advise the following procedure for bathing:

1. Bring your dog into the bathtub or the washing machine. Treats are a fantastic way to start the process off right!

2. Add water to the shampoo to dilute it. Try mixing some in with some water in a bowl, or put the shampoo in a dispenser with some water. Shampoo spreads and suds up better when it is diluted. As most shampoos are thick and concentrated.

3. Spray some warm water on your dog.Taking the temperature with your hand is OK.

4. Give the dog two baths.The shampoo helps remove the filth by binding with it the first time. When you wash your hair a second time, you're actually washing your skin and removing any lingering oil and grime.A loofah sponge to assist in disseminating the shampoo. Remember to pay attention to areas like the belly, armpits, and foot pads. Above everything, strive to make it enjoyable. "You can actually massage the entire dog with your hands. And if you're using warm water, and the dog is in a friendly environment, it should be enjoyable for the dog, according to her.

5. After a few minutes, leave it on and then rinse it off.

6. Rinse thoroughly until the fur is free of all products. While making sure that all of the soap is removed, you should scrub them very well. That's arguably the most crucial factor. Because if you don't altogether remove the soap, it will remain on your skin and aggravate it. It's even worse than not bathing them.

How to Face-Wash a Dog

One of the trickiest steps in bathing your dog is washing his head. Avoid getting water or soap in your dog's eyes, nose, or other delicate body parts. Delaying this step until after the bath and suggests wiping your pet's face with a washcloth.

Your dog's head and face should be gently washed with the washcloth dipped in soapy water. After that, rinse with clear water using a fresh washcloth. Ensure all of the soap is removed from those locations. You should try to avoid the eye area as much as possible when applying shampoo, even if the shampoo is intended to be gentler on puppies' eyes. Have an eye wash on your hands if the shampoo gets in your dog's eyes. Eye goobers on your dog before gently removing them with a toothbrush.

How to Bathe a Canine Water phobic

Even though some dog breeds adore the water (golden retrievers come to mind), many dogs tremble at the mere sound of the bath tap going on. Give your dog lots of praise while bathing him to help combat this. Treats are preferable to praise. When your dog next sees you gathering the dog shampoo, make sure he associates it with good things.

Having a companion hold the dog while you give him a wash is also beneficial. Additionally, begin bathing your dog as a puppy to get him accustomed to the experience.

Tips for After a Bath

First, try your best to towel dry your dog. Then, put a human hairdryer in a medium or relaxed setting or use a hairdryer explicitly designed for dogs. When your dog is drying off. If your dog doesn't shiver excessively or get the chills, let him air dry.

"Every 10 or 15 minutes, run a brush through them as they're drying, and that'll help avoid mats or help separate mats if they have them. Your dog will look and smell better after a bath. Additionally, you will feel good knowing that you did something good for your dog's well-being and appearance.

CHAPTER SIX

Pay attention to your dog's temperament and health.

Before grooming, try to give your pet a good workout. You will only have a little success shaving him if he's acting hyper. To make him more compliant while you're working, "take him for a good walk or get him weary from playing." Be as firm as you can, speak calmly, and have goodies on hand as you groom.

Types Of Exams

There is only one test that works for some. Breeders utilize a few tests to gauge a dog's tracking or Schutzhund's performance. Shelters use temperament evaluations to assess applicants' general disposition and adoption readiness. Others might evaluate a dog's potential as a therapy or assistance dog. Most also assess aggressiveness.

Inquire about the results of any temperament tests your breeder or animal shelter has conducted. Based on what you are looking for, your experience with dogs, and the kind of home environment you can give, they may use these tests to assist choose a puppy for you. For example, an experienced dog owner would better handle a pushy puppy, while a "nosy" breed that is fixated on chasing scents could need a fenced-in yard.

Tests Aren't Always Accurate

Temperament and personality are not fixed characteristics at birth. The early experiences, socialization, growth, and learning consequences all impact your puppy's behaviour.

It may take the dog some time to develop resistance to handling, possessive aggression, territorial vocalization, excessive reactivity, and various forms of dread. When exposed to the stress of an overwhelming environment, shelter pups (especially older ones) you may test may act fearfully or aggressively. However, after leaving the shelter, they may act very differently.

Although you can test puppies as young as seven weeks old, your tests may be more accurate if you wait until they are 3 to 4 months old. The benefit of these tests is that if you can identify the possibility for destructive behaviour via evaluation signs, you can intervene to lessen or eliminate these behaviour with socializing and appropriate training, for example.

Five Puppy Evaluation Exams

These quick evaluations can be done on puppies older than seven weeks.

• Cradle the puppy on its back like a newborn, place a gentle palm on its chest and stare straight into its eyes as the first test for independence. Puppies who consent to this handling are seen as biddable, but puppies that object are more likely to be independent-thinking.

Hold the pup hung under its armpits with its hind legs dangling and stare it directly in the eyes as the second independent-mindedness test. Puppies that comply are thought to have low willpower, whilst those who struggle could want to do things their own way.

- To test a dog's noise sensitivity, drop keys or a tin pan on the ground. Puppies with sound sensitivity have an intense emotional or physical reaction to a sharp or loud sound in the surroundings. The pup shouldn't be cowering or acting irrationally; you want the dog to respond and accept that the sound was made.

- People-friendly test: Watch how the dog responds when a stranger enters the room or when the room is left empty. The puppy either runs to greet or runs away crying. A puppy should be thoroughly acquainted with people by the age of three months.

To determine whether a dog is more independent, prone to attachment problems and separation anxiety, or more calm and easygoing, there is one more test that is useful for evaluating older puppies. In a room with new toys, place the particular puppy with his breeder (or shelter employee) and observe how the dog performs after the person goes. Puppies typically fall into one of three categories:

- Independent: It made no difference to the dog whether the human left or returned. This might indicate a propensity for more independent behaviour, willfulness, or unsuitable bonding.

- Extremely dependent: The dog clung to the human whenever they were there and moaned and ignored toys when they were gone. This could imply concerns with over attachment that could foretell future separation anxiety.

- Moderate: The dog observed the person's entrance and exit but was unperturbed and loved the toys. This denotes a suitable attachment and a laid-back disposition without the need for either coddling or firmness.

CHAPTER SEVEN

Vaccination as a way of grooming a dog

Make sure your dog's immunizations are current if you've newly adopted a dog and are taking it to the groomer for the first time or if you've tried the DIY method and are ready to turn that work up to a professional. To lower the danger of disease transmission between the dog and the groomer and between other dogs visiting the same dog grooming business, dog groomers are legally obligated to check vaccination records for dogs before grooming them.Here's everything you need to know to make sure your dog's first grooming appointment goes off without a hitch.when to have a puppy groomed at a pet spa salon

When Should a Puppy Get His First Bath?

However, bringing them to a groomer benefits your puppy as soon as their vaccinations are current. Some dog owners believe it's best to put off grooming until the puppy is older—waiting until the puppy is about six months old or more extended. Between the ages of 12 and 16 weeks, dogs often have had all the necessary vaccines to visit the groomer.

Early exposure makes it simpler to train dogs to behave appropriately when working with a groomer since it helps them get used to the feeling of being groomed. Due to your puppy's smaller size and the fact that shorter periods will make training more straightforward and less stressful for your dog, early grooming sessions may be shorter. Try to take your dog to the groomer regularly after the initial grooming—every three months or so, but some breeds need more frequent grooming treatments.Vaccinations Required for Grooming Dogs

There is no universal dog vaccination schedule due to the many health concerns and factors that must be considered. Depending on what's best for your dog's health, your veterinarian may have a specific vaccine schedule they advise. No matter what routine you decide on for your dog, it would be best if you had some mandatory vaccinations administered before a groomer would offer services.

These necessary canine vaccinations generally follow a fixed schedule:

Parvovirus and distemper vaccinations are given at 6–8 weeks.

DHPP injection, which includes the vaccines for distemper, parvovirus, parainfluenza, and adenovirus, is given between 10 and 12 weeks. Your dog might be able to go to the groomer for the first time after this immunization.

DHPP booster and rabies vaccination at 16 to 18 weeks.

12–16 months: booster doses of DHPP and rabies

DHPP booster every one to two years.

Rabies booster every one to three years.

Vaccinations must be current on the grooming day, so make sure of that. If your dog's age indicates that the next DHPP vaccination is past due, your groomer will probably insist that you obtain the shot before the grooming appointment.

Being vaccinated against rabies, as well as any additional booster shots or immunizations mandated by local law, should be documented. As established by your local government, you should also make sure your dog has any other vaccinations that are necessary but are not listed above. Your neighbourhood veterinarian can confirm that your dog's vaccination record complies with these regulations.

If your dog is current on his vaccinations, you may bring him in for grooming at any time after 48 hours following the most recent injection. Once a dog reaches adulthood, they only need yearly booster shots

How soon after shots can I groom my dog?

for several vaccines to properly immunize them against diseases. When it's time for your dog to have another booster shot, the veterinary clinic will probably send out reminders if you establish routine care with a nearby veterinarian.

If you take your dog to a new groomer, you should provide the groomer with a copy of your dog's immunization record so they know it is healthy enough to work with. Have these records on hand to prevent last-minute cancellations of appointments owing to uncertainty over your dog's vaccination history.

Additional Dog Grooming Rules

Do you want your puppy to have a positive grooming experience? Before your dog's first appointment, familiarize yourself with crucial dog grooming guidelines to ensure a positive experience for all parties. Typical policies comprise:

Do not take your dog to the groomer 48 hours after vaccination. Following a vaccination, dogs may become agitated or uncomfortable and may experience an adverse vaccine reaction at this time. Bring your dog in for grooming after they have recovered from the vaccination.

While your dog is getting groomed, make yourself reachable by phone. Queries or worries may come up while grooming your dog. These can include your dog's preferences for the haircut style, fears about rashes, or other health issues that surface during the grooming procedure. Have your phone ready and the ringer on for the benefit of your dog and the groomer.

Heed their instructions when the groomer asks you to help with your puppy or leave the office during the grooming visit. It's common for groomers to request that owners leave the office or, at the very least, stay out of view to remove distractions, even though some groomers may ask for your help in relaxing or managing your dog as they get to know your pet.

Grooming your dog is not just a luxury for them. Immunizations are crucial for your dog's health and hygiene, so be sure to keep both appointments.

CHAPTER EIGHT

Conclusion

Assemble your grooming supplies. Once you start grooming your dog, you want to avoid searching for your tools. Before you begin the task at hand, make sure you have everything you need in one location. To find out what you'll need to groom your dog, refer to the "Things You'll Need" section below. First, comb your dog. [1] Most mats can be avoided by searching your dog's coat every day or every other day. For dogs that can mat up, brushing alone is insufficient, contrary to what most literature suggests; the brush will pass over areas where a comb might get caught. The initial step in grooming should always be a thorough combing because any mats will dry and get tighter and harder to handle. Start with the head and work your way down the body. Remember to comb the tail and not scratch the sensitive area under the belly.

If you come across a tangle when combing, try to untangle it with a brush. Be careful to avoid overbrush your dog in one area by doing so for an extended period.

Check if the skin turns red from irritation by peeping underneath the fur.

Short-haired dogs can be brushed with inexpensive items like curry brushes or gloves.

Use more specialist tools to comb and brush medium- to long-haired dogs, such as a steel comb, slicker, pin brush, or undercoat rake.

Whatever you choose must remove loose hair and spread skin oils throughout the coat.

As necessary, give the dog breaks. Avoid overwhelming the dog; any bad associations could make future grooming more difficult. Make the experience enjoyable by occasionally giving your pet breaks, giving praise, food, and pets, and even engaging in a little bit of play. Additionally, this will keep your dog occupied.

This is particularly crucial with a puppy, which can be trained from a young age to endure this much handling effectively.

Cut out mats that are difficult to brush away. When the dog moves, severe matting can pull the skin, making daily life painful for your pet. Depending on how close to the skin it is, you must either cut or shave off a mat if you can't remove it with a brush. If you use scissors, use extra caution to prevent hurting yourself or your pet. To avoid a choppy appearance, try to cut parallel to the direction of hair development.

Bring your dog to a trained groomer if you don't think you can safely remove the mat without injuring him.

Sometimes mats can become so snug against the skin that bacterial illnesses develop there. Visit the vet as soon as possible if you suspect an infection in your dog.

Visual signs of bacterial infection include redness, wetness, and pus secretion in more severe cases. Because it itches, your dog may chew or scratch the area.

Open the canine's eyes. Breeds with white hair or those with big, watery eyes (Pekingese, Pugs, Pomeranians, etc.) may require more upkeep than others in this area. This procedure might only involve cleaning or removing eye lint from the corners of the eyes, depending on your dog. Dogs with long or white hair may require extra care to remove all dirt from the coat because they are more likely to get tear stains. At a pet supply store, you can purchase items designed to remove "tear stains" off white skin.

A healthy eye should be clear and devoid of any discomfort or unusual discharge.

Avoid trying to clip your pet's hair yourself around the eyes because you risk hurting them. Request your veterinarian or groomer.

Clean the ears of your dog. A clean ear will typically contain some wax, but it shouldn't smell in any specific way. Apply some ear-cleaning solution (purchased at a pet supply store) on a cotton round and clean your dog's ears with it. Not too much, or the wipe will drip into the ear. Remove debris and wax from the inner ear by wiping; avoid excessively rubbing, as this could lead to ulcers. Likewise, avoid getting too close to the ear. Wipe the inside of the ear flag if your dog has drop ears like a basset hound because dirt also builds up there. The general rule for groomers is to clean what is visible.

Before applying the ear cleaning solution to the dog's ears, please bring it to body temperature. As you would with a baby bottle, submerge it in a body-temperature water bath.

After cleaning the ear with a damp cotton ball or cloth, gently dry it with another one.

Reward your dog! He could want some comfort because the ears are a delicate body area.

Printed in Great Britain
by Amazon